Paul 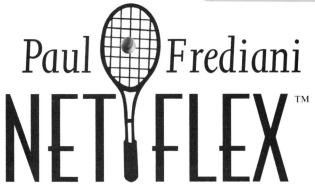 Frediani
NET FLEX™

10 Minutes a Day to Better Play

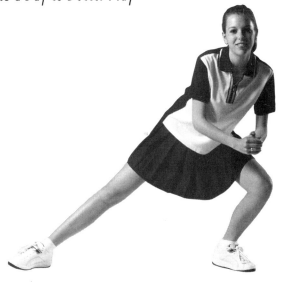

Hatherleigh Press
New York
A GETFITNOW.com Book

Net Flex: Ten Minutes a Day to Better Play
A Getfitnow.com Book

Hatherleigh Press / Getfitnow.com Books
An Affiliate of W.W. Norton & Company, Inc.
5-22 46th Avenue Suite 200
Long Island City, NY 11101
1-800-528-2550

Visit our website: www.getfitnow.com

Disclaimer:

Before beginning any exercise program consult your physician. The authors and publisher of this book and workout disclaim any liability, personal or professional, resulting from the misapplication of any of the training procedures described in this publication.

All Getfitnow.com titles are available for bulk purchase, special promotions, and premiums. For more information, please contact the manager of our Special Sales Department
at 1-800-528-2550.

Library of Congress Cataloging-in-Publication Data
TO COME

Cover design by Lisa Fyfe
Illustrations by Joy Chen
Text design and composition by Dede Cummings Designs

Photography by Peter Field Peck
with Canon® cameras and lenses on Fuji® slide film
Additional photography copyright of Digital Stock, a division of Corbis Corporation.

Printed in Canada on acid-free paper
10 9 8 7 6 5 4 3 2 1

Contents

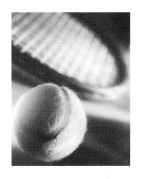

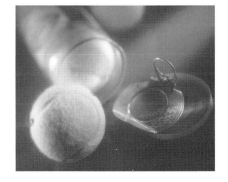

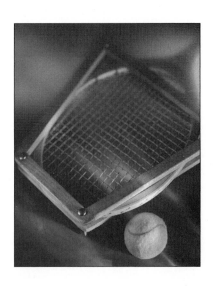

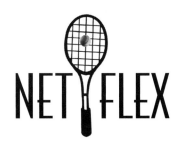

Part I

INTRODUCTION

Welcome to Net Flex! You have just taken a positive step to improve your tennis game. My name is Paul Frediani, and I am a fitness advisor and personal trainer. I create and develop fitness and flexibility programs for everyone from weekend warriors to professional athletes, and the one thing that they have in common is that they all dislike stretching. Why? Because they find it time-consuming, boring, and too complex.

Not anymore. Net Flex is simple, quick, and enjoyable. Follow me and learn how flexibility can increase your power, help you avoid injuries, and keep you in the game.

Net Flex is a ten-minute-a-day flexibility program designed for tennis players of all levels and ages. It is specifically designed to prepare and warm up the muscles used on the court. Such training is called sports specificity.

In addition, I have designed functional stretching for tennis players that can be performed during their everyday living activities. This functional stretching incorporated into everyday tasks is the essence of Net Flex.

The key to developing flexibility is consistency—plain and simple. If you move your body in specific motions, it will respond over a period of time. I am sure you did not pick up your tennis racquet the first time and have a great game. You developed the skill over time, creating muscle memory. To improve your mobility, and hence your game, you need to build memory of certain movements into your joints. But you will not achieve better range of motion in your joints unless you stretch regularly.

Net Flex was developed not only to prepare you in a systematic and easy-to-follow way for your pre-game warm-up, but also, very importantly, to help you find and create ways to add stretching to your life on a consistent basis. What more can you ask for than a program that is enjoyable and effective, yet not time-consuming?

Part II

THE IMPORTANCE OF NET FLEX: WHY STRETCH?

Aren't we all interested in maintaining independence in our lives through mobility? None of us want to be slaves to our injuries, which can become chronic, forcing us to give up our active lifestyle. With just a little effort and an awareness of our daily living habits, we can avoid most common tennis injuries. Many shoulder and knee injuries are a direct result of inflexibility, weak muscles, and poor postural habits.

As we get older and become less active, we naturally lose flexibility, and this increases the risk of injury to our joints, tendons, and muscles. A consistent stretching program can reduce soreness and increase power in your game.

BENEFITS OF STRETCHING

- Reduces risk of injury

- Increases range of motion

- Increases body awareness

- Improves circulation

- Reduces muscle tension

- Reduces soreness

- Relaxes and relieves stress

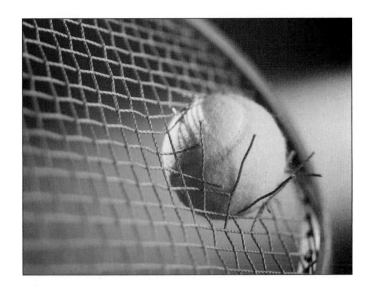

THE WRONG WAY TO STRETCH

"Hey! Get out of the way! Watch out!" **How often have you almost been brained by a flying racquet, or by someone swinging a racquet around to get warmed up? I can't think of a worse way to stretch. Your muscles are cold and your grip is not yet warmed up. It is a good way to invite injury to yourself and someone else.**

Stretching staticly—stretching, holding it, then moving to the next stretch—feels real good, doesn't it? Your muscles get nice and relaxed. Unfortunately, they will be in for a big shock if you stretch this way before playing tennis. Asking your muscles to relax, then swinging your racket at full speed or sprinting across a tennis court just doesn't make sense. Static stretching should be done after your game.

Dynamic stretching is what should be performed before you play. Stretching dynamically means moving while you stretch. Dynamic stretching prepares the muscles for the actions they will be asked to perform in a sport-specific setting, and at the same time it warms your body temperature in preparation to play the game.

THE SCIENCE OF NET FLEX

Power is force produced over a distance per unit of time. In tennis, power is the result of a chainlink summation of coordinated movements of your entire body. If any of these three elements can be increased—force exerted, speed (unit of time at the face of the racquet during the backswing), or range of motion (flexibility)—the result will be a more powerful groundstroke.

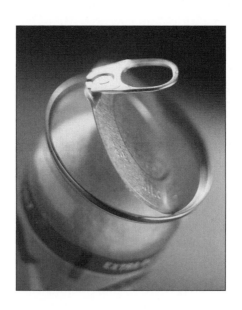

STRETCHING MYTHS

● Myth 1—It's too time-consuming. There's no way I can fit it in my busy schedule.

You do not need to take time out from your day to stretch. You can start a flexibility program before you even get out of bed, while working in the office, or even in the car.

● Myth 2—Flexibility training is for professional athletes only. It is much too complex to do alone. I would have to hire a personal trainer and spend a fortune.

Net Flex is as easy as one, two, three. Complex fitness programs just don't work. If you have read this far, you're smart enough to follow this program. Save your money to buy a new racquet.

● Myth 3—I will never be flexible.

You will never be flexible if you don't stretch. It may be true that you'll never do splits, but short of major injuries, you can significantly improve your range of motion. The aging process naturally shortens and tightens your muscles. Flexibility training can help reverse that process.

Myth 4—I don't need to stretch everyday. I just stretch well once a week before I play.

Stretching once a week will do this for you: absolutely nothing. To increase your range of motion or improve flexibility, you need to stretch ten minutes a day. Consistency is the key.

Myth 5—Stretching is so boring!

Think about adding 20 to 40 mph to your serve. Boring? I think not. Professional tennis players are adding that much power to their game simply because they have discovered the indisputable benefits of stretching. Lack of flexibility can make your groundstroke backswing short and narrow, reducing power to the stroke. Same goes for your service motion. So think about that when you start to yawn. What can be more boring than sitting home tending to your injuries? Reduce flexibility and you will increase your potential for serious injury.

Myth 6—I am too old to stretch.

It's never too late to begin a flexibility program. There is no better time than right now! If you want to be successful, avoid injuries, and have the satisfaction of a better game, stretching is the key. What are you waiting for? There are people running marathons in their 70s and 80s. The great John Glenn is back in space. Let's get busy! Let's stay active! Just a few minutes a day and you will see how much more limber you feel after only a few weeks.

IMPROVING YOUR FLEXIBILITY

Stay with the Net Flex program. Give yourself time to stretch daily and you will be amazed at how quickly your body will respond. Do not over-stretch or give up if you miss a day. After a while, stretching will become as natural a part of your day as brushing your teeth.

Try to be aware of activities that can hinder your progress. Some of the simplest everyday tasks can hurt you in the long run—sitting with your legs crossed, carrying a bag slung over your shoulder, working hunched over at your desk. You can improve your flexibility by removing bad posture habits.

Water, water, water. We lose flexibility as we get older largely due to the lack of movement needed to transport fluids to our joints. Drinking plenty of water helps replenish these necessary fluids, keeping our muscles flexible. Try to avoid caffeine and alcohol, or at least increase your water intake after drinking these beverages to reduce dehydration.

Remember that you can be very flexible in your lower body while still having a very tight upper body. Tailor your Net Flex program to address your body's individual flexibility needs.

Part III

FLEXOLOGY

The following areas of the body are important to an overall flexibility program for tennis players. Net Flex will address each of these areas and how they relate to your strokes. The serve, volley, forehand groundstroke, and backhand groundstroke each constitute a complex action using many muscle groups together in a synchronized chainlink movement.

The "flexspots" are the muscle groups that work together to give you a fluid stroke. Spend a little more time stretching the areas that are particularly tight. It is important when you do the Net Flex stretches to follow the program in the order it is designed.

Neck—During your serve, you are constantly putting stress on your neck. Warm up by relaxing the neck and preparing it for the impact and rotation of the serve.

Upper Back and Shoulders—Increased flexibility in the upper back and shoulders will allow for greater rotation and range of motion in your serve's backswing, resulting in more speed and power.

Upper Arms—Focusing on this area will help the rotation of your serve by giving you greater range of motion through your elbow joints and shoulders.

Lower Back and Trunk—Definitely the most crucial area to keep flexible and healthy, the lower back is the center of your groundstrokes. Every time you squat down to hit a low ball or bend over to pick up a ball, you are lifting half your body weight. All tennis strokes rely heavily on back stabilization and movement.

Inner and Outer Hips—Want to generate power? You've got to turn your hips. This is true in almost all sports. (It is said that Joe Louis, the great heavyweight boxing champion, would turn his hips so crisply when he punched that you could hear his trunks snap against his thigh.) The hip stretch is also essential for hip weight transfer during your groundstrokes.

Hands and Wrists—Prepare and warm up your hands and wrists for impact. Stretching these areas will help you avoid the nagging injury tennis elbow and give you better control of your racquet.

Hamstrings and Quadriceps—Not only will tight hamstrings and quadriceps fatigue and tighten your legs, it will also effect your lower back and hips, considerably restricting your coverage of the court.

Calves, Achilles Tendon, and Ankles—Constantly pivoting and changing direction on the court can easily fatigue and cramp your calves. Stretching before and after your game will help prepare your muscles for the task of omnidirectional play and eliminate soreness. Achilles tendonitis, a common tennis injury, can quickly become chronic. It can best be avoided by frequently stretching these areas well.

MECHANICS OF THE SERVE

Let's take a look at the mechanics of a serve and at how improving your flexibility can create more power. The serve is a complex motion, requiring the use of many joints in your body. The more joints used in a movement, such as throwing a football, swinging a bat, or throwing a punch, the more power your body is able to deliver. The power of the serve doesn't come from the arm—it comes from the legs and torso rotation.

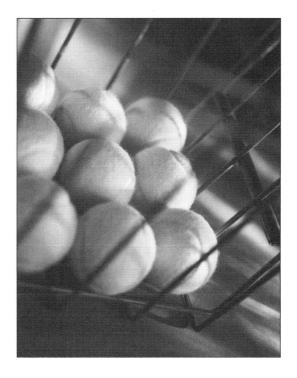

1. You begin the serve with your knees slightly flexed and your weight on your front leg (your left leg, if you're right-handed). The leg, butt, and back muscles are engaged. The abdominal muscles should be tight to protect the lower back.

2. As you throw your toss, your left arm goes up, your right arm goes behind your back, and your weight shifts to your back leg. You need optimum flexibility in your shoulder (specifically, the rotator cuff).

3. As you bring your racquet up and forward to make contact with the ball, your leg, shoulder, upper back, and arm muscles are engaged. (And, depending on the style of serve you choose—e.g., flat or slice—you may also be rotating your wrist and forearm at impact.) It is the forward motion of your entire body that creates the power, not just your arm muscles.

MECHANICS OF THE GROUNDSTROKE

You're facing the net when the ball is returned to you. Keeping your knees bent, you now must pivot your torso right or left for either a forehand or backhand groundstroke. For this, you need flexibility in your back, hips, and abs.

After running to the ball, you position yourself with your weight on your back leg and your knees bent, according to the height of the ball. For topspin, you want to hit the ball from low to high, so keeping your knees well bent can assist you in achieving that motion—as much as your shoulder and arm muscles. (For backspin, or a "slice" shot, you want to keep your back strong while hitting from high to low. This requires a stable back and strong and flexible shoulders.)

After you've struck the ball with a topspin groundstroke, you want to follow through on your stroke so that your racquet finishes high. This, again, requires flexibility in your torso.

While forehands and backhands both require leg, hip, back, and shoulder strength and mobility, forehands engage the biceps more and backhands engage the triceps more.

Volleys at the net do not require long backswings or follow-throughs on their swings, but their "punching" motion requires strong back muscles to support the arms and flexibility in the arms and legs for reaching for those quick jabs.

By increasing the range of motion in all your joints and surrounding muscles, and by increasing the strength in your abdominal muscles to deliver power to your legs, hips, and upper torso, you will be able to deliver more power to your strokes.

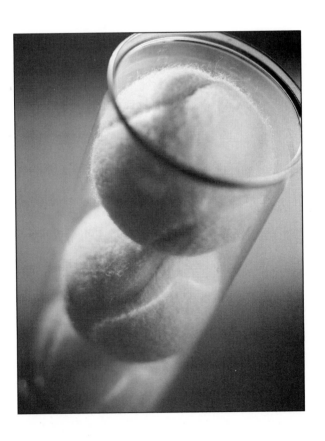

Part IV

The Net Flex Program

THE STRETCHES

Stretching is not a competition. What you do not achieve today may come tomorrow. However, you will never know if you don't stay on path. Often times, people that are naturally talented in a certain activity never achieve greatness because they quit at the first obstacle. Commitment is all it takes.

In this program, we will focus on two types of stretching—static and dynamic. Static stretching requires simply holding a stretch for 10 to 20 seconds. We're going to start with static stretching so that you get used to each different stretch and recognize the muscles involved. With that accomplished, you can move on to dynamic stretching, which involves actively moving into a stretch and holding it for three to five seconds, then repeating the motion five times. With each motion, the stretch gets deeper and deeper. This doesn't mean "bouncing" or "jerking" into a stretch—it means simulating the kind of motions you are most likely going to make on the court during play. Such stretches incorporate lunging, for example.

The best stretching to do before playing tennis is dynamic stretching, because it also serves as a warm-up to your game. Once you've performed each of the following stretches statically and feel comfortable doing them, perform them dynamically before your game. Repeat each stretch five times, then try to move quickly from one stretch into the next. This will get your heart pumping, your muscles warmed up, and it will make the stretching program go quickly so you can get into your game.

Before we begin, let's keep in mind some simple points:

1. Always breathe.

2. Never hold your breath.

3. Maintain good posture.

4. Never bounce or jerk.

5. Never force or strain your muscles when you stretch.

6. Maintain consistency.

7. Stay in touch with your body and focus on the muscles being stretched.

8. Never over-stretch (i.e., pushing into a painful stretch).

9. Consult a doctor before beginning any flexibility program.

10. Smile and relax.

Did you know that tightness is often a sign of muscular weakness? Flexibility and strength training go hand in hand. Identify your weakness and improve your strength. Conversely, did you know that stretching can also help strengthen weak muscles? True!

STATIC STRETCHES

1. YES AND NO

Nod your head "Yes" by bringing your chin to your chest, then back up to the neutral position. Start the "No" movement by facing forward, turning your head slowly to the left until your chin is over your left shoulder, then slowly to the right until your chin is over the right shoulder. Neck exercises should be done gently. Repeat this exercise eight times.

Muscles used: Neck muscles.

Result: Prepares and warms up the neck for shoulder rotation and the impact of hitting the ball.

Tip: Add half moon rolls, which are chin rolls from one shoulder to the chest to the other shoulder. Be careful not to extend the neck backward.

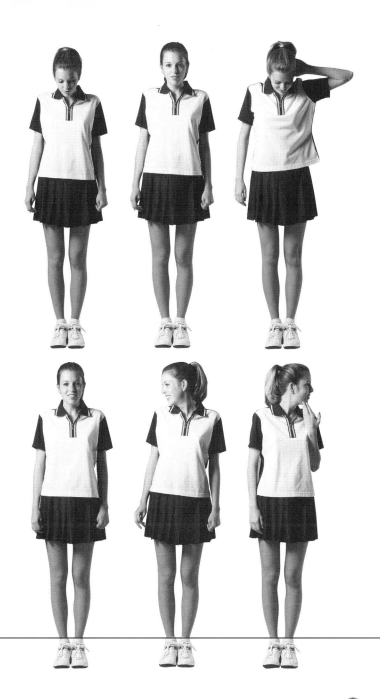

2. SHOULDER ROLLS

Lift your shoulders to your ears—forward, down, back, and up. Reverse directions, and repeat the motion eight times both ways.

Muscles used: Shoulder muscles.

Result: Warms up the shoulders and prepares the neck for the impact of the swing.

Tip: Great stretch to relieve neck and shoulder tension.

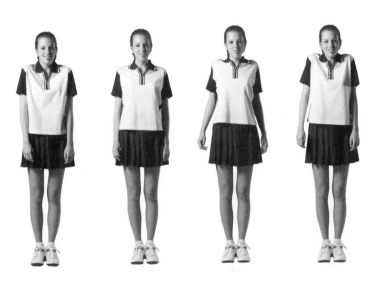

3. BACK SCRATCHERS

Reach one elbow up toward the ceiling and your hand behind your neck and toward the opposite shoulder. With the other hand, assist the stretch by gently pulling back on the elbow. Repeat eight times on both sides.

Muscles used: Backs of arms, shoulders, and back muscles.

Result: Improves serve, backswing, impact, and follow-through.

Tip: Bend at the waist to increase the stretch.

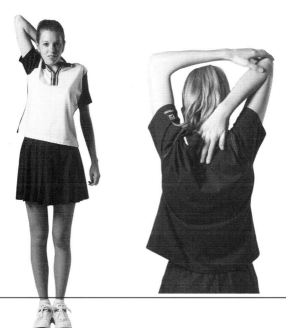

4. BACK STRETCHER

Keeping your shoulders down, stretch your left arm across your chest, and gently pull your left arm toward you with your right hand. You can add more intensity by turning your torso. Switch arms and repeat eight times on both sides.

Muscles used: Upper back, arms, and shoulder muscles.

Result: Improves backswing and follow-through.

Tip: Keep your shoulders down and away from the ears.

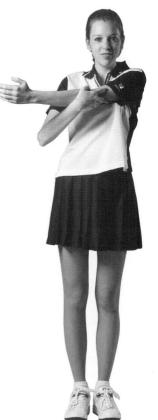

5. TREE HUGGER

With your feet shoulder width apart, pretend you're wrapping your arms around a big tree. Keep your chin to your chest as you contract your stomach muscles. You will feel this stretch from your tailbone to the top of your head. Repeat ten times.

Muscles used: Full back and spine stretch.

Result: Helps backswing, downswing, and impact.

Tip: Be sure to keep your abdominal muscles tight.

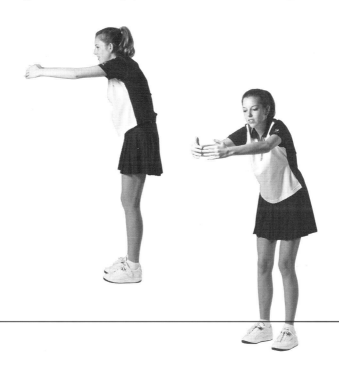

6. ROOSTER CROWS

Interlace your fingers behind your back. Squeeze your shoulder blades together as you stick out your chest, pressing your hands backward. Look up toward the ceiling, contract your butt, and stretch the front of your shoulders and chest. You want to keep your chest open to achieve a greater range of motion in both your back and forward swings. Combine with the tree hugger stretch, and repeat ten times.

Muscles used: Chest, front of shoulders, and upper back muscles.

Result: Improves backswing and follow-through.

Tip: A slight arch in the lower back will increase this stretch. When stretching, remember your ears and shoulders are mortal enemies. Keep your shoulders down!

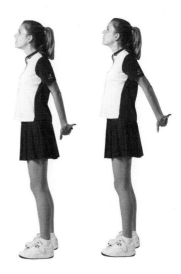

7. BYE-BYES

With your arms out to the sides, bend your forearms up from the elbows 90 degrees with your palms facing forward. Then, rotate your forearms, pressing your palms down. Repeat eight times.

Muscles used: Rotator cuffs.

Result: Benefits the serve, backswing, downswing, impact, and follow-through.

Tip: Keep your shoulders stable and only rotate the arms. Work smoothly and slowly. Add dumbbells for more intensity.

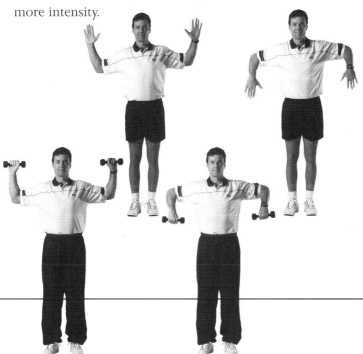

8. EMPTY BOTTLES

This is another great shoulder warm-up. Keep your arms straight and point your thumbs toward the floor. Start with your hands near your thighs and lift them to shoulder-height, repeating eight times.

Muscles used: Rotator cuffs.

Result: Improves serve, backswing, impact, and follow-through.

Tip: Keep shoulders down and back.

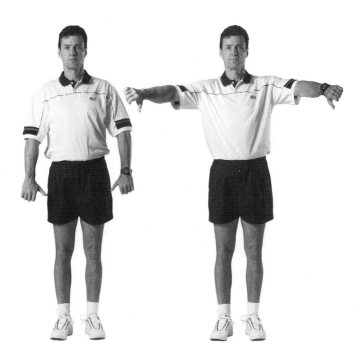

9. PEACH PICKERS

With your feet shoulder width apart and your knees slightly bent, keep your stomach tight as you reach one hand toward the ceiling and the other toward the floor. Stretch your waist and shoulders as you alternate hands. Repeat the motion eight times. Advanced—For a more intense stretch, reach further and bend more from the waist.

Muscles used: Waist and shoulder muscles.

Result: Improves serve, backswing, and follow-through.

Tip: Deepen your knees by bending and reaching laterally to increase your stretch.

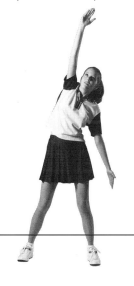
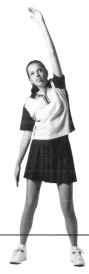

10. WILLOW TREE

Cross your feet, interlace your fingers, and reach the palms of your hands toward the ceiling. Advanced— Bend from the torso from side to side four times. Switch feet position and repeat.

Muscles used: Forearms, arms, fingers, shoulders, waist, hips, and legs.

Result: Improves serve and backswing and prepares the upper body for impact with the ball.

Tip: Keep your abdominal muscles contracted and your butt tight.

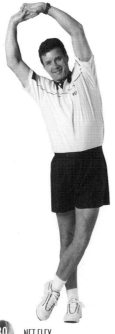
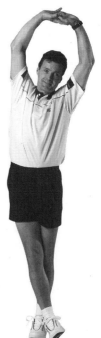

11. WRIST ROLL WITH FINGER SPREADER

With your fingers loose, roll your wrists clockwise, then counter-clockwise five times. Advanced—Press the tips of your fingers together as you separate your palms, stretching your fingers apart.

Muscles used: Hand and wrist muscles.

Result: Helps serve and prepares the hands and wrists for impact with the ball.

Tip: If needed, repeat during play to help alleviate post-game soreness.

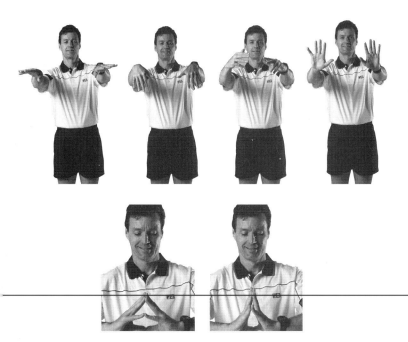

12. FOREARM FLEX AND STRETCH

With one arm extended in front of you, gently press your fingers down with your opposite hand, palms inward. Repeat the motion pulling your fingers back with your palms facing outward. Perform this stretch five times on each hand.

Muscles used: Forearm muscles.

Result: Improves serve and prepares the forearms for impact with the ball.

Tip: This stretch, in combination with strengthening exercises, will help prevent tennis elbow.

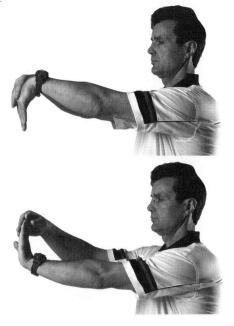

13. HELICOPTERS

Stand with your feet shoulder width apart and your arms extended out to the sides. Keep your face and hips forward as you rotate your torso to the left and right, keeping your arms straight. Advanced—Twist your torso as you reach your right hand to your left pocket and your left hand to your right pocket. This stretch is excellent for torso rotation. Switch sides and repeat ten times.

Muscles used: Waist and torso muscles.

Result: Improves your serve, backswing, and follow-through.

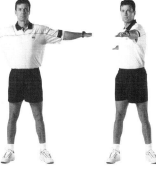

Tip: Start slowly and keep your face forward, increasing your rotation as you progress. Be sure your abdominal muscles are tight and your knees bent.

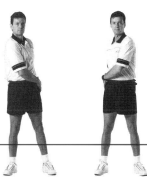

14. HULA HOOPS

Don't laugh, this is a great way to warm up through the hips. Think it's easy? Well, it was when you were twelve years old. With your hands on your hips, rotate your pelvis in circles. Repeat ten times in each direction.

Muscles used: Hips and waist muscles.

Result: Helps serve, backswing, and follow-through.

Tip: Start with small circles and gradually increase their size.

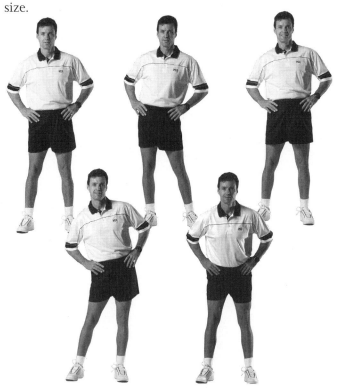

15. HAMSTRINGS

Bend forward at the waist, keeping your stomach tight and your back flat. Do not bounce. Stay where you can feel the stretch and hold for ten seconds, repeating twice. Tight hamstrings = tight back = tight strokes.

Muscles used: Back of leg muscles.

Result: Improves serve, backswing, impact, follow-through, and movement around the court.

Tip: It is not how far you go, but how consistent you are with the stretches that will improve your flexibility.

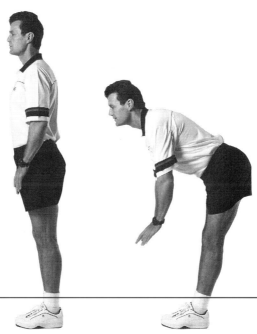

16. QUADRICEPS

Standing straight, grab your foot or ankle behind you and pull your heel to your butt. Try to keep your knees together. Hold onto a chair or wall if you need additional support. Hold for ten seconds, and repeat twice with each leg.

Muscles used: Quadricep muscles.

Result: Helps backswing, impact, and follow-through.

Tip: By pressing your hips forward, you will increase the stretch in the front of your hips.

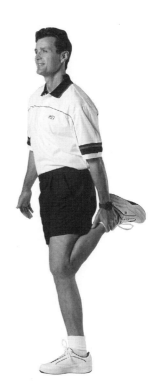

17. CALVES AND ACHILLES TENDONS

Lots of quick, sudden movements can easily fatigue your lower legs. Standing with one foot in front of the other, keep your feet facing forward and press your rear heel on the ground. Feel the stretch in your calves for ten seconds, repeating twice. Advanced—Slightly bend your rear knee for an advanced Achilles tendon stretch.

Muscles used: Calf muscles and Achilles tendons.

Result: Improves follow-through, prevents Achilles tendonitis, and prepares your calves for impact and movement around the court.

Tip: Be careful not to bounce when doing this stretch.

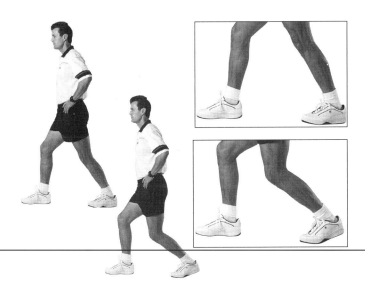

18. KNEE AND ANKLE ROTATORS

Place your hands on your knees and slightly bend your legs. Keep your knees and feet together as you rotate your knees clockwise and counter-clockwise eight times.

Muscles used: Knee and ankle muscles.

Result: Serve, backswing, impact, and follow-through are improved.

Tip: Preparation is crucial for this area. The volley—and any shot you have to jump for— puts a lot of stress on the knee joints. Start with small circles and work toward larger ones.

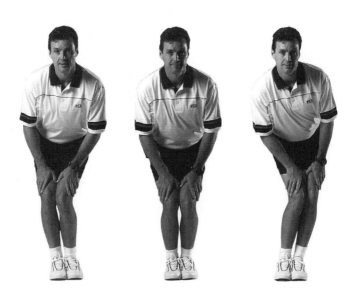

19. INNER THIGH

Stand with your feet more than shoulder width apart and rest your hands on your hips or thighs for support. Keep one leg straight while bending the other leg and hold for eight seconds. Switch legs and repeat four times. Advanced—For a more challenging stretch, place your hands on the floor between your legs.

Muscles used: Inner thigh muscles.

Result: Helps backswing and prepares the leg muscles for impact with the ball. It's important to stretch the groin well.

Tip: If this stretch is too difficult, try the seated butterfly stretch (see page 52).

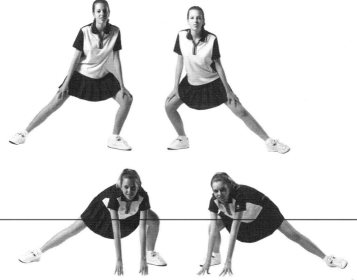

20. HAY BALERS

With your feet shoulder width apart and your palms together, stretch your arms straight out in front of you. Drop your hands to your left foot and then up over your right shoulder. Switch sides and repeat ten times.

Muscles used: Lower and upper legs, butt, waist, torso, shoulders, and arms.

Result: Improves serve, backswing, impact, and follow-through.

Tip: Hay balers are the final touch to complete our warm-up, combining all the stretches in a synchronized movement. Add one to three pound weights on each hand to increase the intensity of this exercise.

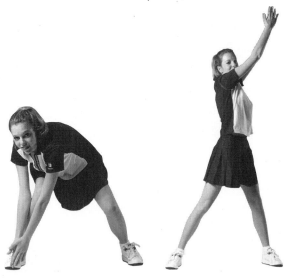

21. GLUTE STRETCHES

Lie on your back on the floor. Raise one knee up to your chest. Keep rotating the angle of your knee. For example, raise your left knee to your left shoulder, then position the knee closer to your mid-chest, then closer to your right shoulder.

Muscles used: Hips, butt, and torso.

Result: Improves flexibility when retrieving low balls and making lunges in any direction.

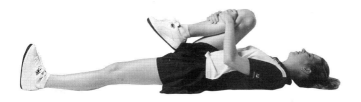

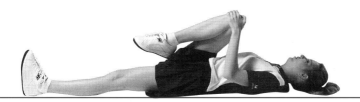

DYNAMIC STRETCHES

All the stretches above can and should be done dynamically. When you are ready to do them dynamically, add the following lunges:

1. SIDE LUNGE

Start by rocking back and forth, then touching each toe. Reach to one side, then the other. Then, turn more completely, pivoting on your feet.

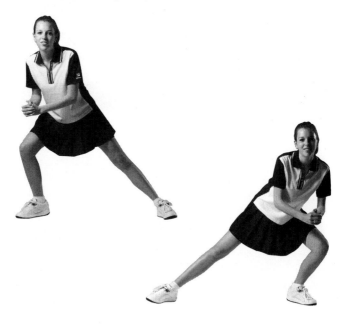

2. FORWARD LUNGE

Lunge forward with
one leg and reach
down with both
arms. Do five lunges
with each leg.

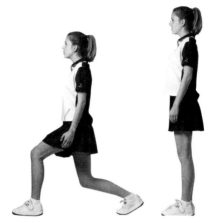

3. BACK LUNGE

Face forward with your legs together, then pivot on one
foot, turning back to lunge, and face forward again.

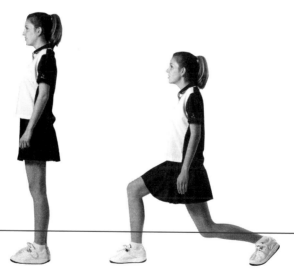

POST-GAME DOUBLES FLEX

While pre-game dynamic stretching warms your muscles, helps avoid injuries, and prepares your body for the movements of tennis, post-game static stretching alleviates soreness and keeps your muscles from snapping back tighter than they were before the game.

Assisted stretching is the best type of stretching you can achieve—if done properly. The key to couples stretching is communication. The flexor is the one assisting the person being stretched, who is the flexee. Be sure to maintain your breathing pattern and not hold your breath. Never force or bounce your partner's limb into a stretch. Hold stretches for 10 to 20 seconds. Be aware of your partner's posture while stretching—also be aware of your own. What good is it if you stretch your partner but kill your back?

1. LATS

Flexor stands
behind flexee
and places hands
slightly below
flexee's elbow
and assists the
flexee's arm as it
reaches for the
opposite
shoulder.

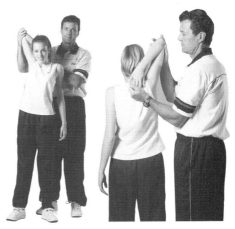

2. UPPER BACK

Flexor stands behind flexee
and places one hand on
flexee's back while the other
hand reaches in front and
gently assists the flexee's arm
from above the elbow move
across the flexee's body.
Remind the flexee to keep the
shoulders relaxed.

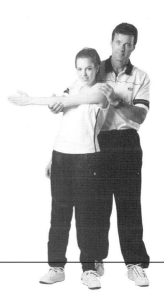

3. SHOULDERS

Flexor stands behind flexee. The flexee interlaces hands behind back. Flexor very gently lifts arm away from body.

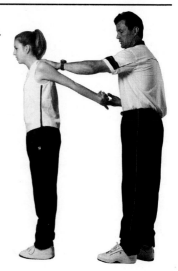

4. HAMSTRINGS

Flexee lies on his or her back and lifts one leg to feel a stretch. Flexor places one hand behind flexee's heel and one hand on the thigh and adds a gentle stretch. A tight hamstring equals a tight back.

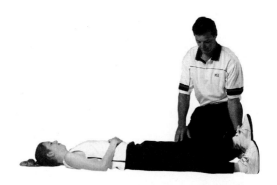

5. CALVES

In the same position as the hamstring stretch, place the hand that was behind the heel on the ball of the foot, and gently add pressure as you point the toes upward.

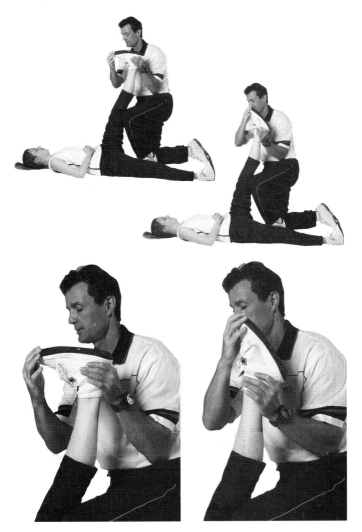

6. ADDUCTORS

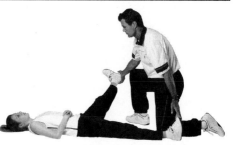

Flexee lays on his or her back on the floor, placing a rolled towel or small pillow under the head if stress is felt in the neck. Flexor lifts flexee's leg off the floor and gently moves it to a point where the flexee feels the stretch. Make sure the flexee's leg is straight and that the toes of both feet are pointing to the sky and the hips stay firmly on the floor.

To get a deeper groin stretch, the flexee can bend the leg being stretched 90 degrees at the knee, while the flexor gently applies pressure to the bottom of the foot.

7. ABDUCTORS

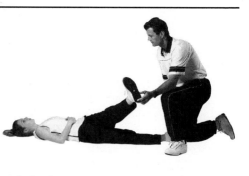

The flexee lies on his or her back on the floor. The flexor stands on the opposite side of the leg being stretched. Lift the leg to be stretched, making sure the knee is straight and that both hips remain on the

floor. Bring the leg being stretched across the leg on the
floor until the flexee feels the stretch. It's important to
keep the non-working leg stable with its toes pointing
up. This keeps the hips stable.

8. IT BAND

The IT band is prone to chronic overuse injury. It can
sideline many players if it's not stretched. The flexee lies
on his or her back and bends the non-working leg and
places its foot on the outside of the working leg. The
flexor places one hand on the bent knee, the other hand
under the heel of the leg being stretched, and gently lifts
and stretches the leg to the opposite side.

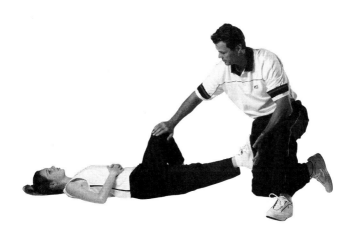

EVERYDAY SEATED STRETCHES

These stretches are a wonderful addition to your Net Flex workout and an excellent way to stretch in your spare time. The following stretches can be done while lying in bed or watching television, to help stretch your back and hips—two key power areas in tennis. Although these stretches may not be possible to do on the court, you should find time to practice them during the day.

1. INDIAN SITS

This is a great outer hip stretch. Start by sitting on the floor with your legs crossed, leaving both feet on the ground. Incorporate a back stretch by placing your hands on the floor in front of you. Lower your chin as you walk your hands forward, letting your chest fall to your knees. This is a wonderful multi-purpose exercise, which stretches your hips, butt, shoulders, and back. Alternate sides and repeat. Advanced—Increase your hip stretch by sitting with one foot over the opposite knee.

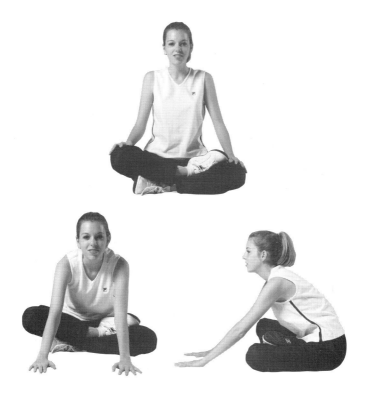

2. CHILD POSE

Sit on your heels, drop your chest to your knees, and reach your hands out in front of you. A great relaxing stretch, this exercise stretches your ankles, legs, butt, and back.

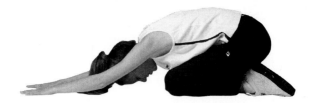

3. BUTTERFLY

Sit with the soles of your feet together and your knees out to the sides. Hold your ankles as you gently press your knees apart with your elbows. Be careful not to bounce.

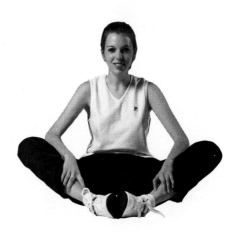

4. CORKSCREWS

Sit with your left leg straight and cross your right foot over your left leg. It is important to keep your back straight. Do not slouch! Place your right hand behind you, and your left arm outside your right leg. Turn and look toward your right hand. Be sure to pay attention to your breathing. Without changing feet position, turn and face the other direction. Hold each of these positions for 30 seconds. Repeat with the opposite leg.

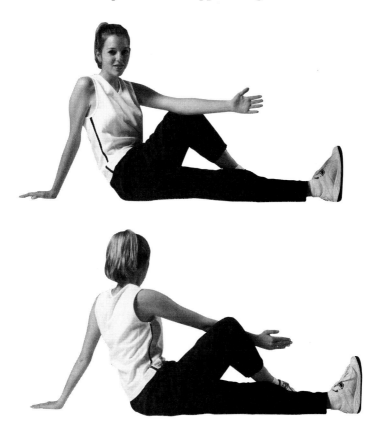

5. ABDOMINAL AND BACK STRETCH

Lie on your stomach and lift your chest up on your elbows. Flex your abdominal muscles as you stretch your back. Advanced—Lift your entire upper body up on your hands. This is a much more intense stretch. It is not recommended for those recovering from lower back injuries.

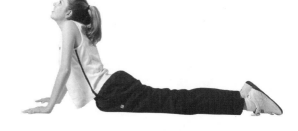

6. LOWER BACK STRETCH

Lie on your back and bend one knee, while keeping the other leg straight. Hold the shin of your bent knee to your chest. Repeat with the opposite leg. Advanced—For added intensity, hold both shins to your chest.

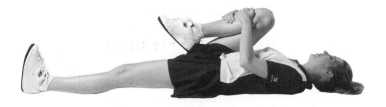

7. TINKERBELL

Lying on your back, bend your right knee over the left, keeping your left leg straight. Pull the right leg across with your left hand and look in the opposite direction of the stretch. Reach your right hand out to the side and repeat with the opposite leg. Advanced—Keep your right leg straight as you cross it over your left leg. Hold both arms out to the sides. Repeat with the opposite leg.

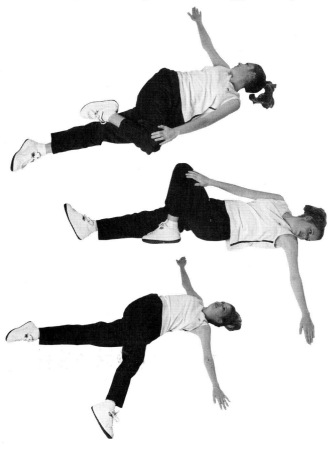

THROUGHOUT THE DAY

You may say, "The Net Flex program is great, but how am I going to stretch during the week? I hardly have time to eat breakfast and kiss the family goodbye. I just don't have time for a flexibility program."

This is the beauty of Net Flex. You can practice your flexibility routine anywhere—at home, in the car, or at the office. Just do a few minutes at a time and you will achieve long-term results.

Now let's incorporate these stretches into our daily lives. You will see how easy it is to stretch as you do your everyday tasks, and how quickly your flexibility will increase.

In Bed. Do these stretches before you get out of bed in the morning and your back will love you. Bring one knee to your chest, hold for ten seconds, and alternate knees. Then, bring both knees to your chest for ten seconds. Fold your knees over to one side, then

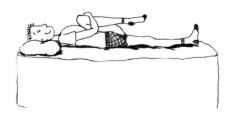

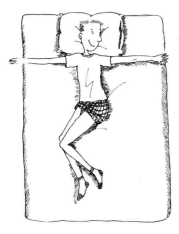

the other side, holding for ten seconds each. Be sure to keep your shoulders flat on the bed. As you increase in flexibility, move smoothly from one position to the next. These stretches will warm up, stretch, and prepare your back and spine for the day!

Rise and shine. Give yourself a big hug, stretching your upper- and mid-back. Hold one arm across your chest and hug it toward you with the opposite hand. Alternate arms, stretching the shoulder muscles.

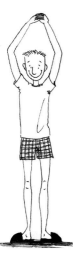

From either a seated or standing position, interlace your fingers and lift your hands over your head, pushing your palms away from you. This stretches your forearms, shoulders, and ribcage. This exercise can be increased by gently leaning over to one side, stretching your waist. Be sure to keep your abdominal muscles tight while doing this stretch.

Time to shower. A nice hot shower is an excellent opportunity to warm up and stretch. Start by letting the hot water hit the back of your neck, relaxing your upper back and neck muscles. Slowly do half circles, letting your chin roll from one shoulder to the other. Repeat approximately six times.

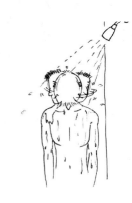

Now that your back is warmed up, do a few tree huggers. Let the water run down your upper- and mid-back. Hold each stretch for ten seconds. Continue to stretch your back by adding a few back scratchers.

Turn and face the water, letting it warm your chest muscles as you do six rooster crows. You have just gotten a great upper body stretch in no time. Shower everyday, stretch everyday—see the difference it makes!

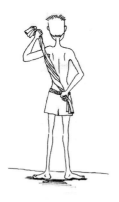

Toweling off. Grab a towel at both ends, bringing one hand over your head and one behind your back. Reverse the motion and rotate your hands. This is a wonderful way to stretch your rotator cuffs and keep your shoulders healthy.

Stand with one foot forward, bending your rear knee and keeping your front leg straight while you towel off. To increase this stretch, wrap the towel around your forward foot and gently pull towards you. This exercise increases the strength and flexibility of your calves and Achilles tendons.

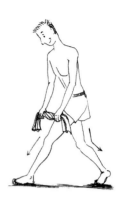

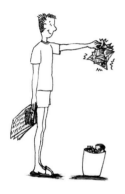

Reading the paper. You do it every morning! Take this time to also strengthen your hands and forearms. After reading a section of the paper, take a sheet in one hand and slowly crumble it into a tight ball. This is a lot harder than it seems. Try getting up to four sheets per hand.

Getting dressed. Putting on a shirt is something we do everyday and it can be a great stretch for our shoulders, ribcage, and arms. As you put one arm through your shirt, reach as far as you can toward the sky, and repeat with the opposite arm.

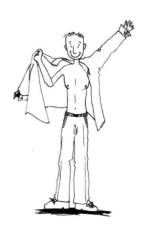

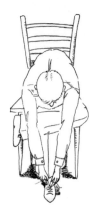

Putting on socks and shoes.

While seated, cross one ankle over the opposite knee and feel the stretch in the back of your legs and butt as you lean over to put on your sock. Reverse leg position and put on the other sock. Then slip on your shoes. Go down on one knee as you tie your shoe,

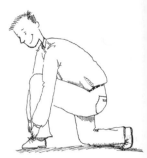

stretching the front of your hip and your back leg.

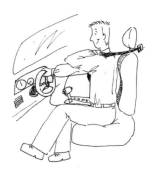

Sitting in the car,

waiting for it to warm up. Keep your right hand on the steering wheel and reach your left hand across

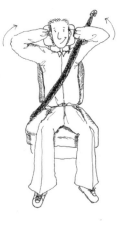

your body to the back of your seat. This really opens up your back and shoulders. Repeat on the opposite side.

Interlace both hands behind your head and reach backward, stretching both your chest and back.

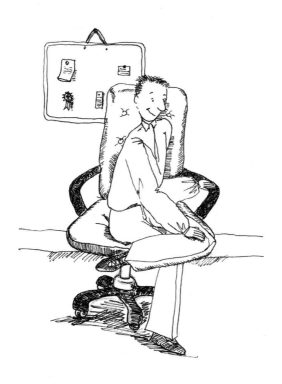

At the office. For many, sitting at the office all day can make us tight and often tense. Sitting with our legs crossed for hours at a time while hunched over our desks, does nothing to promote flexibility. However, taking just a few minutes a day, you can easily increase your well-being and flexibility. There is an old Italian saying, "Chi va piano va sano e lontano," meaning, "He who goes slow, goes safely and far." A little every day will get you results!

Sit with your left ankle over your right knee. Keeping your spine straight, place your right hand on your left knee, and turn your torso to your left. In the same seated position, turn your torso to the right by placing your left hand on the outside of your right thigh. This is a great spine stretch! Continue by placing both hands on your thighs and gently lower your chest toward your knees, stretching your butt, back, and thighs. Reverse feet position and repeat.

Sit with your feet flat on the floor and slowly drop your head between your knees, letting your hands fall to the floor. You will feel this stretch in your lower back and butt. While in this stretch position, remember to breathe deeply into your lower back, filling your lungs and slowly letting tension release with each exhale.

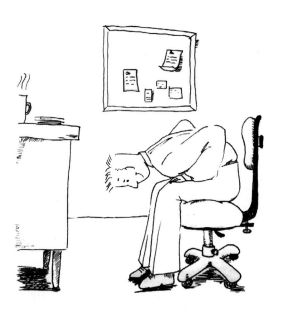

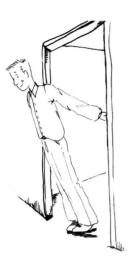

Grab both sides of the doorway with your hands at shoulder level. Walk forward until you feel the stretch in your arms. This exercise is great for your chest and shoulder muscles.

The following stretches can also be done seated at your desk:

- Yes and No

- Peach Pickers

- Willow Tree

Part V

Net Flex Injury

Hot Spots and Prevention

By Nick Anthony

While muscle overuse is a common cause of injury for professional tennis players, weekend players' injuries are most often a result of improper form, muscle weakness, and lack of flexibility.

You will notice the back, abs, and hips are included in the following injury prevention exercises. These areas are sometimes referred to as the power zone. In any sport that requires the motion of throwing or swinging, this part of the body stabilizes and generates power from your trunk to your torso.

INJURY HOT SPOTS

Elbows/Wrists/Forearms—Gripping the racquet often results in impact and overuse injuries.

Shoulders—The shoulders are the most common area injured in any sport that involves throwing or swinging.

Back—The serve and groundstrokes can cause major strain from the neck to the lower back.

Hips—If your hips are tight, you will not generate rotation power; and if your back is tight, your hips will overcompensate, causing overuse injuries.

Feet/Ankles—Sudden stops and direction changes can cause soreness in the front of your ankle and the soles of your feet, and also may result in shin splints.

TENNIS ELBOW AND HAND STRENGTHENING

Tennis elbow is a nagging, painful injury that, if not properly cared for, can become chronic. A form of tendonitis, tennis elbow is a result of wear and tear over time. To care for this injury, there is one word you should burn into your memory—RICE. No, not the kind you get with Kung Pao chicken. R.I.C.E. is an acronym for:

Rest—to prevent further injury and relieve stress from the area of discomfort.

Ice—reduce swelling by decreasing circulation to the area.

Compression—bracing or wrapping the injured area to reduce expanding and swelling.

Elevation—to decrease the amount of blood and fluid to the irritated area.

Depending on its severity, tennis elbow can take six weeks or longer to heal. It is important to see a doctor for a proper diagnosis. Once the inflammation is reduced, you can incorporate stretching and strengthening exercises. The biggest mistake most people make is not resting long enough. Playing again too soon can result in re-injury and further damage. The key to recovery is REST.

Wouldn't it be even smarter to avoid this injury instead of rehabilitating it? Let's look at some simple and effective stretching and strengthening exercises.

Hand Squeeze — Spread open your hand, then make a tight fist. Continue to open and close your hands, working up to 50 times.

Hand Squeeze With Resistance — Using a pliable rubber ball or old tennis ball, squeeze and release your fist. Keep a ball handy at your desk and do this exercise throughout the day.

Sand Gripping — Fill a bucket with sand and shove your hand in up to your wrist. Keep your hand in the sand as you open and close your fist. This is one tough exercise, but it will give you great results!

Let's begin where the rubber hit the road—the hands, wrists, and forearms. Any weakness here will surely result in tennis elbow. Strengthening the hands will give you the control needed to improve your game and avoid injury.

As mentioned earlier, a simple way to incorporate hand-strengthening exercises into your day can be done while reading the newspaper. Taking one sheet at a time, use one hand to crumple the page into a tight ball. Do three or four sheets a day and you will notice an increased hand grip. When you swing, your wrists and hands work to generate power and control the tennis racquet.

1. RUBBER BAND STRETCHES

Place a rubber band around your fingertips and extend your fingers as you try to open your hand.

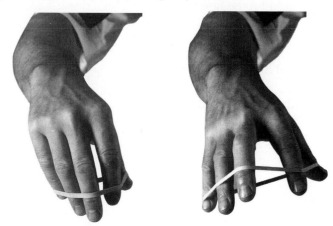

2. BALL SQUEEZES

Holding a ball, squeeze your hand together into a tight fist. Start with softer balls and move up to more resilient balls as your strength increases.

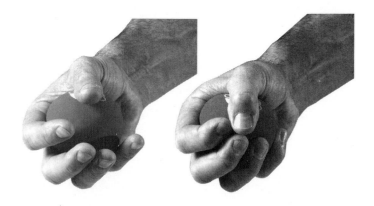

3. RACQUET PRONATIONS AND SUPINATIONS

Hold a racquet in one hand out in front of you. Rotate the racquet so that your palm is facing up, then down. Repeat with both arms.

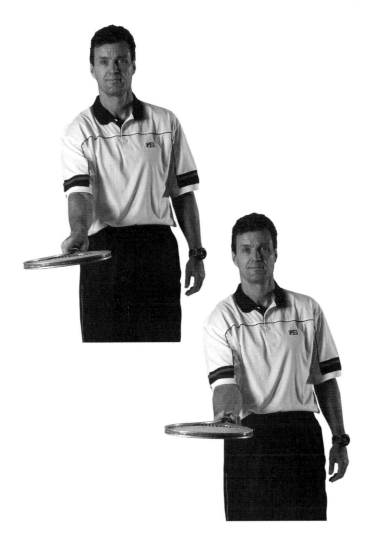

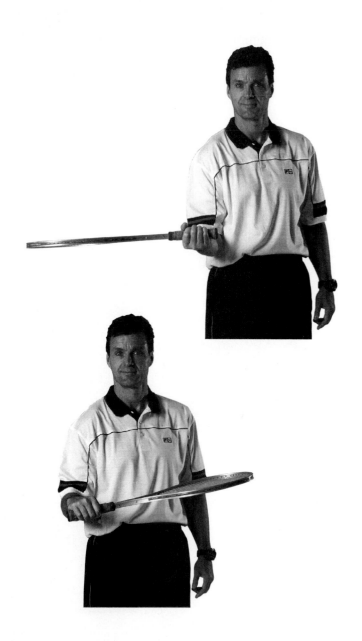

4. TOWEL ROLLS

Hold a towel with both hands out in front of you. Twist your hands in the opposite directions as if you were wringing out the towel.

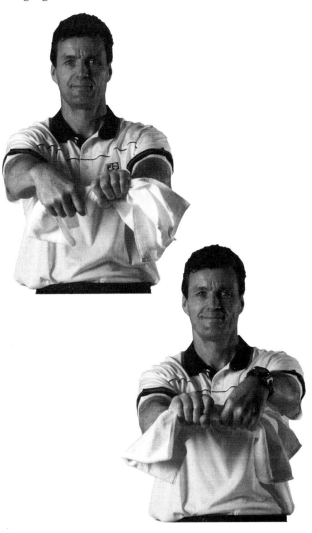

5. FINGERTIP PUSH-UPS

Lay on your stomach with your elbows bent and your hands by your sides. Push off your fingertips and toes to raise your body up. Hold the position for a few seconds and slowly lower your body back down to the ground.

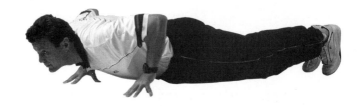

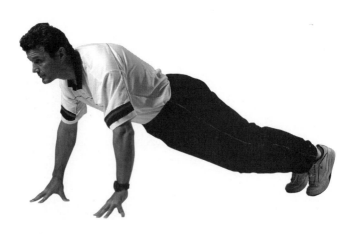

SHOULDERS

Because of its structure, the shoulder is the most mobile joint in the body. Its support is dependent upon balanced muscular flexibility and strength. Unfortunately, the sport of tennis can place large quantities of shearing force on the shoulder joints and the muscles that protect these joints, namely the rotator cuffs. Because of these forces, a flexibility and strength imbalance and extreme forces surrounding the joint can lead to numerous shoulder injuries. While it is important to stretch and strengthen the rotator cuffs, for overall shoulder health, it is important to develop flexibility in the chest and strength in the back and deltoids, allowing for maximum shoulder strength throughout an entire range of motion.

Tips

1. Always stretch after performing these exercises.

2. Use a pillow or rolled up towel to support your head if you feel neck strain.

3. Work in slow and controlled movements.

4. Use a full range of motion.

1. SUPINE SHRUGS

Lie on your back on a bed, couch, or bench. Allow one shoulder blade to "hang" off the edge. Extend your arms as high as possible and then lower them beyond the level of the bench. For an additional challenge, practice this exercise while holding dumbbells.

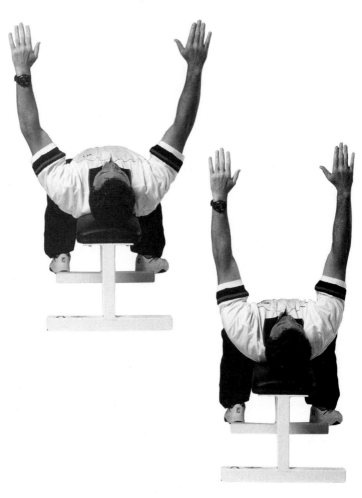

2. ALPHABET WITH TOWEL

Place a towel against a wall or door and hold it with your hands five to six inches apart. Extend your arms and lean against the towel at a 45-degree angle. Spell out the alphabet in capital letters with big sweeping motions while leaning forward with your hands against the towel.

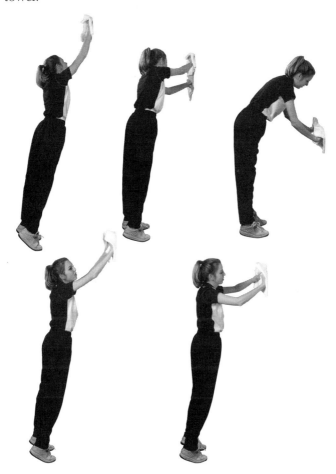

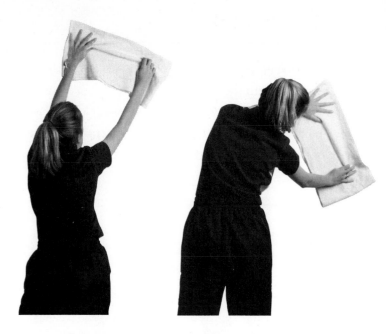

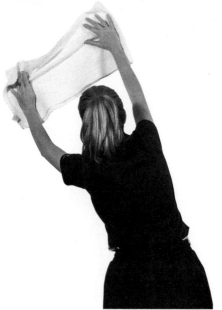

3. BYE-BYES

With your arms out to the sides, bend your forearms up from the elbows 90 degrees with your palms facing forward. Then, rotate your forearms,

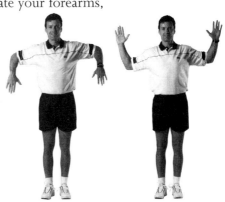

pressing your palms down. Repeat eight times. Keep your shoulders stable and only rotate your arms. Work smoothly and slowly.

4. SOUP CANS

Use the same movement as the empty bottles stretch described on page 28, but add resistance. Do three sets of ten, starting with soup cans and working up to three-pound weights. Keep your arms straight and point your thumbs toward the floor, with your pinkies up toward the ceiling. Start with your

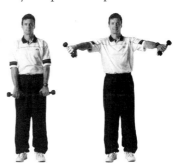

hands near your thighs and lift them to shoulder-height, repeating eight times.

5. EXTERNAL ROTATIONS

Lie on your side with your legs together and your knees bent. Place your bottom arm behind your head for support and your top arm at your waist, bent 90 degrees. Rotate your forearm from your stomach straight up and repeat on the other side. Start with three sets of 20, using one- to three-pound weights and work up to five pounds.

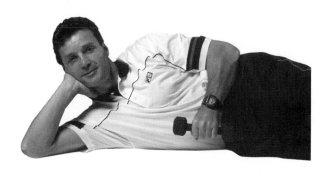

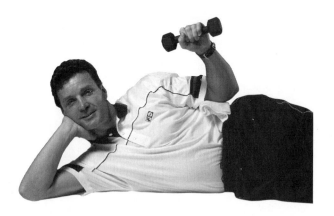

6. INTERNAL ROTATIONS

Lie on your side with your legs together and your knees bent. Rest on your shoulder with your top arm at your hip, and your bottom arm bent 90 degrees. Rotate your bottom arm from your stomach to the floor and repeat on the other side. Start with three sets of 20 using one- to three-pound weights and work up to five pounds.

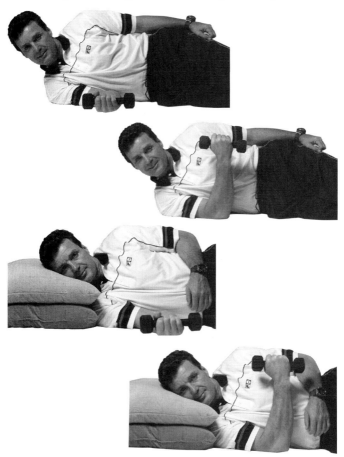

7. LATERAL RAISES

Stand with your knees slightly bent and your feet slightly apart. Holding three- to five-pound dumbbells at your sides, raise them laterally to shoulder-height. Do three sets of 10 to 20 repetitions.

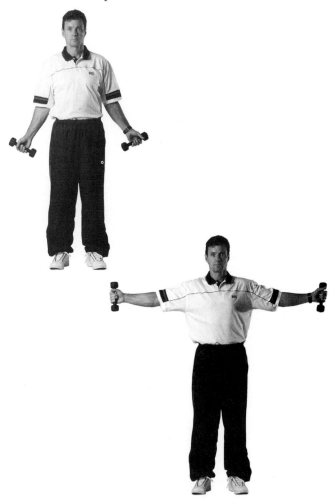

8. REAR DELT RAISES

Stand with your knees slightly bent and your feet slightly apart. Bend over so that your upper body forms a 90-degree angle at your hips. Holding three- to five-pound dumbbells with your arms hanging down toward the ground, raise your arms out to the side and up to shoulder-height. Do three sets of 10 to 20 repetitions.

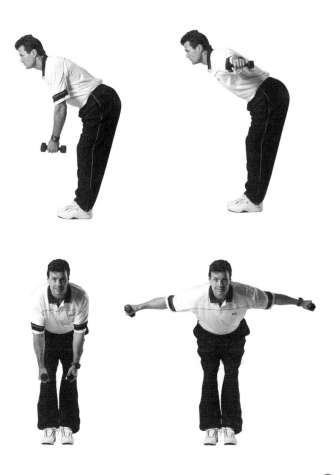

9. FORWARD RAISES

Stand with your knees slightly bent and your feet slightly apart. Holding three- to five-pound dumbbells at your sides, raise them forward and up to shoulder-height. Do three sets of 10 to 20 repetitions.

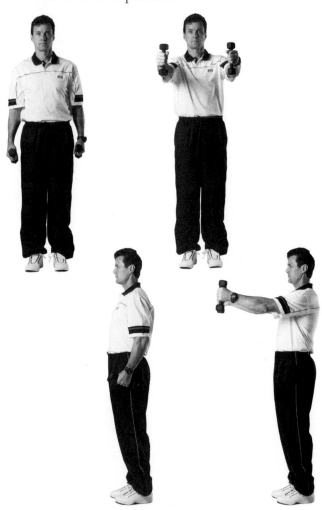

ANKLE AND LOWER LEG

For many tennis players, the ankle is the most frequently injured body part. While there are many supporting structures around the ankle to assist in joint stability, twists are a very common occurrence for many sports enthusiasts. Ankle injuries range from slight sprains to more severe injuries resulting in lengthy rehabilitation programs. Flexibility and strength in the calves and ankles, as well as proper footwear, are major considerations for ankle support and health. Here are some exercises to develop joint stability, strength, coordination, and balance for the ankles and lower legs.

1. LEG SWING

Stand on one foot with your knee bent and your eyes closed. Extend your opposite leg out in front of you, behind you, and then to your side, returning to center after each movement. Repeat ten times with each leg.

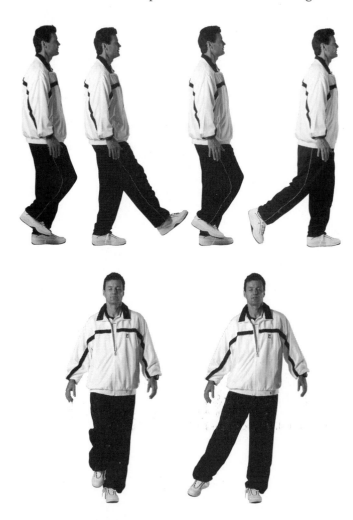

2. FOOT SHIFTS

Stand beside the baseline or sideline. Shift your weight to your toes and swing your heels across the line. Shift your weight to your heels and swing your toes over the line. Now both feet should be across the line. Continue to shift back and forth to either side of the line, repeating eight to ten times.

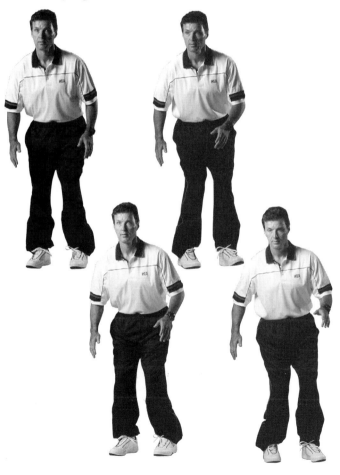

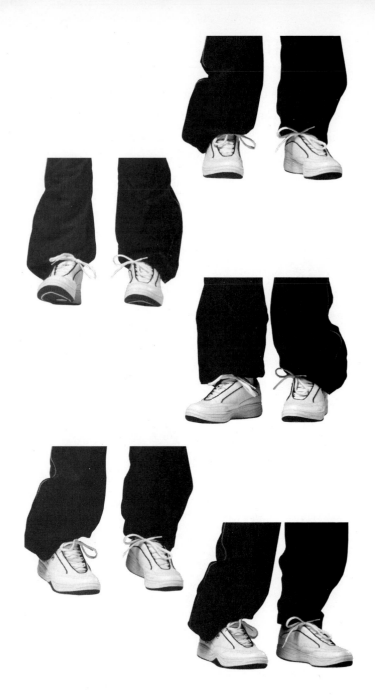

3. CALF RAISES

Stand straight with your feet together and your arms at your sides. Slowly lift your heels so you are supporting your weight on the balls of your feet. For a more advanced workout, cross one foot behind the other ankle and lift onto only one foot.

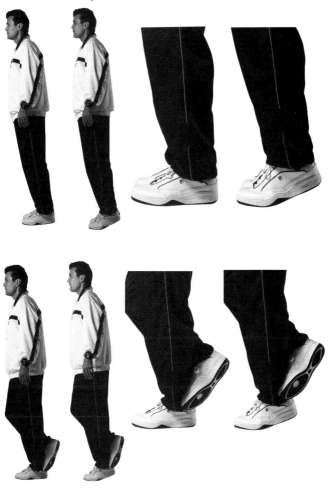

4. HEEL WALKS

Stand straight and lift your toes off the ground, supporting your weight on your heels. Hold your arms out to the sides or in front of you for balance as you walk forward on your heels.

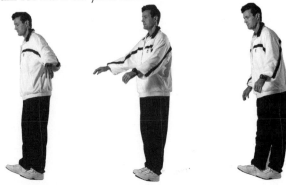

5. WALKING LUNGES

Lunge forward and dip your hips toward the floor three times while in the lunge position. Raise up and lunge forward with the opposite leg, repeating the dips. Do three sets of ten for each leg.

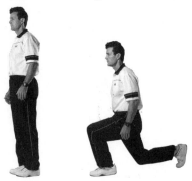

KNEES AND UPPER LEG

Proper footwear, cardiovascular conditioning, flexibility, and proper skill development are important elements of conditioning the knee. To properly protect the knee, it is essential to strengthen the quadriceps, outer and inner thighs, hamstrings, and calves.

1. BODY WEIGHT HALF-SQUATS

Stand with your back straight and your feet shoulder width apart. Slightly bend your knees as you squat, mimicking the motion of sitting in a chair. Be sure to keep your knees aligned over your toes.

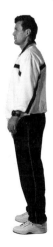
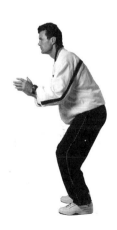

2. GOOD MORNINGS

Stand with your feet shoulder width apart. Hold a broomstick at each end behind your neck. Keeping your legs straight, but not locked, bend over, sticking your butt out behind you. This exercise is a terrific hamstring stretch.

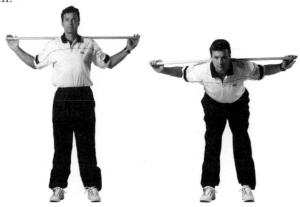

3. LUNGES

Stand with one foot in front of the other with your arms at your sides. Bend your legs, lowering your back knee close to the floor.

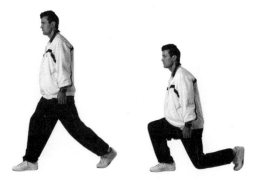

4. TWISTS

Face straight ahead with a wide stance and slightly bend your knees. Turn right by rotating your hips to the right as you drop lower into your stance. Try to keep your right foot pointing forward as you pivot your left foot. Repeat on your left side. This exercise stretches the groin, knees, ankles, and thighs. Repeat 10 to 12 times.

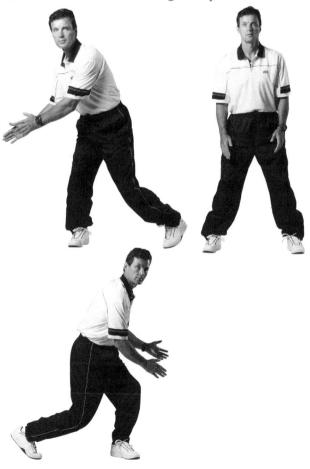

5. LATERAL LUNGES

Facing forward, take a giant step to one side as you hold your arms out to the sides or in front of you for balance. Repeat on both sides. For a more advanced exercise, as you lunge to one side, reach your arms down in front of your extended foot.

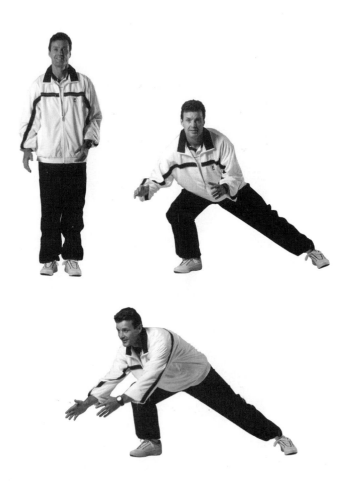

LOWER BACK

The back takes on such a tremendous amount of stress during the serve, groundstrokes, and volley that it is no wonder the lower back is a major source of injury for tennis players. Before engaging in a back strengthening and stretching program, it is important to consult your doctor. The back is a complex area. Problems can arise from stress, poor posture, and certainly poor mechanics of the serve or groundstrokes.

To maintain and condition your lower back, it is essential to keep it strong and flexible. The following are back strengthening exercises. They should be done in conjunction with abdominal exercises. Strengthening your abdominal muscles is an essential part of maintaining an overall healthy and strong back. The abdominal muscles help stabilize the back, while the obliques rotate your torso during your swing. No back conditioning program is complete without abdominal exercises.

1. SUPERMAN

Lie on your stomach and extend your arms in front of you. Lift your chest and arms off the ground.

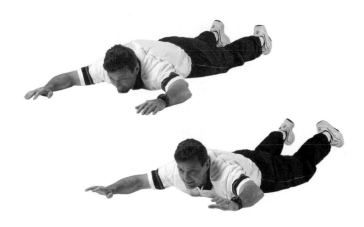

2. LOIS LANE

Lie on your stomach with your hands under your chin. Keep your legs on the floor as you lift your hands and elbows.

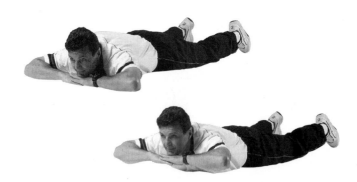

3. SWIMMER

In the same position as the superman stretch, lift your right arm and left leg. Repeat with the opposite arm and leg.

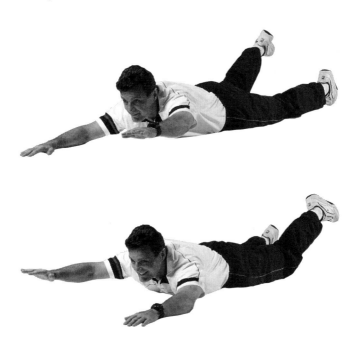

Tip: Holding your knees to your chest is a great way to give your back an overall stretch after exercising.

Seated stretches that add flexibility to your back:

- Indian Sits

- Child Pose

- Butterfly

- Corkscrews

- Abdominal and Back Stretch

- Lower Back Stretch

- Tinkerbell

Back strength and wellness are not only affected by power and flexibility in the back muscles, but are also influenced by flexibility and strength in other muscle groups as well, which affect movement and posture. Proper strength in the abdominal muscles, thighs, hamstrings, groin, and glutes can affect hip alignment and range of motion, which are crucial components of a good overall back.

4. CORE HOLDS

Lie on the ground on your stomach. Slide your elbows underneath your chest so they are even with your nipples.

Interlock your fists and raise your body up on your toes and elbows. Stay as stiff as a board and hold the position for 20 to 30 seconds.

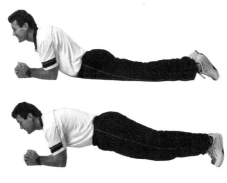

5. SIDE CORE HOLDS

Lie on the ground on your side. Slide your elbow

underneath your side until your bicep is perpendicular to the floor. Raise your body up on your elbow and foot, staying as stiff as a board. Hold for 20 to 30 seconds and repeat on both sides.

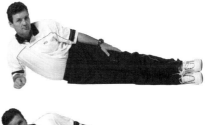

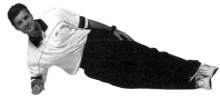

6. REVERSE CORE HOLD

Lie on the ground on your back while supporting your upper body weight on your elbows. Raise your body up on your heels and elbows, keeping your legs and back as straight as possible. Stay as stiff as a board for 20 to 30 seconds.

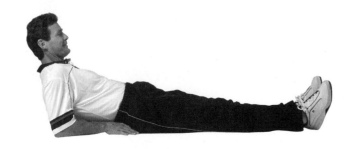

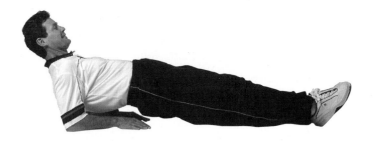

ABDOMINAL EXERCISES

1. STANDARD CRUNCHES

Lie on your back with your knees bent. With your hands behind your head, contract your abdominal muscles and lift your shoulders off the floor. Be careful not to pull on your neck.

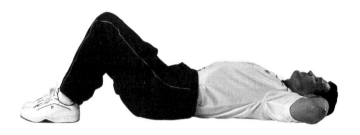

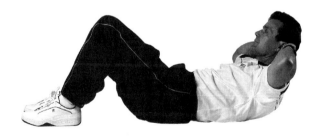

2. REVERSE CURLS

Lie on your back with your knees and feet in the air, and place your hands on the floor at your sides. Lift your hips off the ground and tilt your pelvis up toward your chest. Do not bounce or jerk. Cross your feet for additional comfort. Advanced—With your hands behind your head, lift your hips, shoulders, and head.

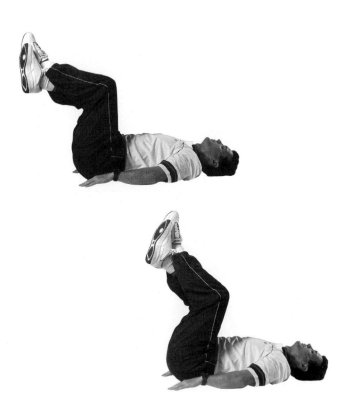

HIPS

The most important part of the power zone, strong and flexible hips will keep you in the game and prevent nagging strains. Fortunately, we have many opportunities throughout the day to stretch our hips. Putting on your socks is a great way to work the sides of your hips, lacing your shoes works the front, and bending over while seated at your desk works the inner thighs.

Here are a few simple thigh and hip strengthening exercises:

1. SCISSORS

Lie on your back with your legs straight, and lift one leg up in the air. Repeat with the opposite leg.

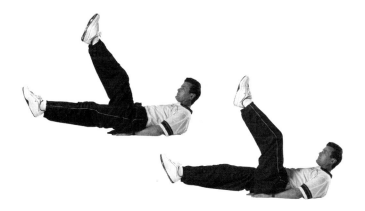

2. INNER THIGH

On your side, cross one foot over the other leg and lift the straight leg six inches off the ground. Repeat on both sides.

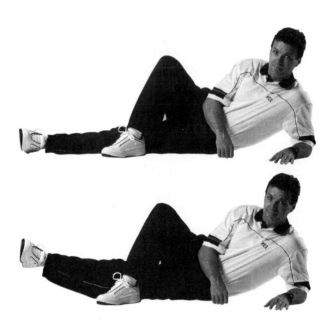

3. STANDING SQUATS

Stand with your feet shoulder width apart. Keep your heels solid on the ground. Drop your butt back as though you were sitting in a chair. Keep your chest high and shoulders back as you try to keep your butt level with your knees.

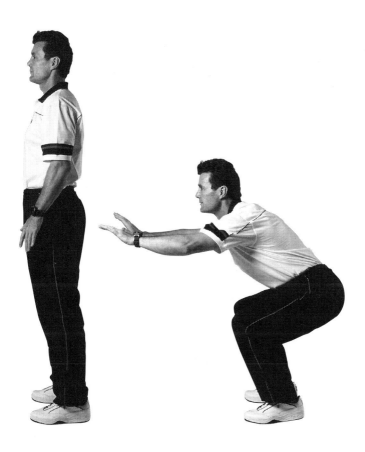

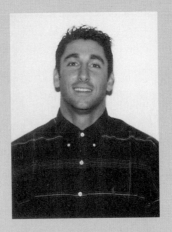

Nick Anthony received his Masters Degree in Exercise
Science from Arizona State University where he worked
with members of the track and wrestling teams as well
as the dance department. He served as a speaker of the
World Scientific Congress of Golf at the University of
St. Andrews and San Diego Golf Academy instructor
educational programs. He has extensive experience
as a strength and conditioning coach with the NFL
and ATP Tour players. He is also a member of the
National Strength and Conditioning Association
and is a consultant for Men's Health magazine and
www. eteamz.com Website.

Part VI

Conclusion

Net Flex was developed out of necessity. As my tennis playing clients rolled in on Monday mornings complaining of muscle weakness and soreness after playing a few sets of tennis on the weekend, I encouraged them to stretch before and after every game.

The response I always got was, "Of course I stretch. Everyone stretches before the game. That's nothing new. Everyone knows the benefits of flexibility training and how it improves your game." So, if they were stretching, why were they always so banged up and sore? So I asked them how they stretched. The response was always the same. "Oh well, I . . . uh, you know, uh, . . . do some of these and then I swing the racquet around, and . . . uh, you know, loosen up."

It was pretty obvious that they didn't have a handle on what they were doing, and that they probably picked up most of what they did from what they saw other players doing on the courts.

It was apparent they had no systematic approach to stretching that they could follow in a safe and effective way.

I developed Net Flex so tennis players could understand and perform stretches in a simple and clear manner. It is just as important for tennis players to continue their stretching everyday to increase flexibility and range of motion in a progressive matter. Net Flex not only improves your game, but also leads to increased body awareness and well-being. You can achieve results, so what are you waiting for? When it comes to stretching, there's never an excuse not to do something.

In health and fitness,
Paul Frediani

MEET THE AUTHOR

An educator for the American Council of Exercise, Paul's interest in fitness began when he was twelve years old, surfing the chilly waters in San Francisco. His interest in sports and fitness led him to compete in open ocean swims, long distance running, and triathlons. He won the San Francisco Golden Gloves and the Pacific Coast Diamond Belt Light-Heavy Weight Boxing Championships. Paul is certified by the American Exercise College of Sports Medicine and is a medical exercise specialist. He is affiliated with Equinox Gyms in New York City, a fitness advisor for Getfitnow.com, and President of BoxAthletics, a fitness training company.

Crunch® Fitness Series

Through the country Crunch® is synonymous with the ultimate in fitness and exercise. From New York to LA, Crunch Fitness Centers have helped hundreds of thousands of Americans get in shape and stay in shape. With their unique lifestyle approach to fitness and their philosophy of "no judgements" on your lifestyle, Crunch is the choice of men and women who want to exercise their right to fitness.

Crunch and Hatherleigh are proud to announce the next three books in the *Crunch Fitness Series*. Each book in the series is specifically designed to meet the lifestyle demands of today's Americans — the harried business executive who spends her weekends on the road, the father of the bride who has to look good in a tux, the soccer mom who just doesn't have time for the gym, young people, old people, couch potatoes and bodybuilders.

Everyone will benefit from the Crunch expertise and their team of fitness specialists.

Crunch is a major national chain of fitness centers. Their brand is widely recognized through a daily television exercise show on ESPN and through their videos and fitness apparel. Their upscale, user-friendly gyms are located in New York, Los Angeles, San Francisco, Miami, Chicago, and Tokyo.

Also available in the
Crunch Fitness Series:

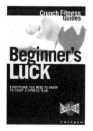 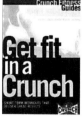 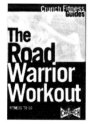

Beginner's Luck
Get Fit in a Crunch
The Road Warrior Workout

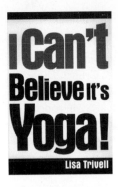

I Can't Believe It's Yoga!

It's Yoga — American Style

Lisa Trivell, Photographed by
Peter Field Peck

A popular form of exercise and fitness conditioning,
yoga combines stretching and breathing to tone the
body, relax the muscles, and relieve tension. The
numerous benefits of yoga can easily be added to
anyone's daily fitness routine.

For many, though, yoga is seen as being both too
difficult and too different to try. *I Can't Believe It's
Yoga* addresses this perception problem by
presenting a yoga based fitness program which is
easy to accomplish.

In *I Can't Believe It's Yoga*, Lisa Trivell, an experienced
yoga instructor transforms even the reluctant
skeptic into an avid fan. Utilizing the most basic yoga
exercises, the results are incredible!

ISBN 1-57826-032-9 / $14.95

Available in bookstores everywhere, order toll free at 1-800-906-1234 or online at getfitnow.com.